CLINICAL APPROACHES TO TACHYARRHYTHMIAS

edited by

A. John Camm, M.D.

Volume 3

CLINICAL APPROACHES TO TACHYARRHYTHMIAS

edited by

A. John Camm, M.D.

St. George's Hospital Medical School
London, United Kingdom

Volume 3

Risk Assessment of Ventricular Tachyarrhythmias

by

Mark H. Anderson, M.D.

Department of Cardiology
Hammersmith Hospital
London, United Kingdom

**Futura Publishing
Company, Inc.**
Armonk, NY

Library of Congress Cataloging-in-Publication Data

Anderson, Mark H., M.D.
   Risk assessment of ventricular tachyarrhythmias / by Mark H.
Anderson.
      p.   cm. — (Clinical approaches to tachyarrhythmias ; v. 3)
   Includes bibliographical references and index.
   ISBN 0-87993-612-6
   1. Ventricular tachycardia—Risk factors.   I. Title.   II. Series.
   [DNLM: 1. Tachycardia, Ventricular—epidemiology.   2. Risk
Factors.   WG 330 C6403 1993 v. 3]
   RC685.T33A53   1995
   614.5'9128—dc20
   DNLM/DLC
   for Library of Congress   94-23609
                                                                     CIP

Copyright © 1995
Futura Publishing Company, Inc.

Published by
Futura Publishing Company, Inc.
135 Bedford Road
Armonk, New York 10504-0418

LC #: 94-23609
ISBN #: 0-87993-612-6

Every effort has been made to ensure that the information in this
book is as up to date and as accurate as possible at the time of
publication. However, due to the constant developments in
medicine, neither the author, nor the editor, nor the publisher
can accept any legal or any other responsibility for any errors
or omissions that may occur.

Printed in the United States of America.
This book is printed on acid-free paper.

Foreword

When all is said and done, cardiac tachyarrhythmias account for considerable distress and untimely death. The arrhythmias may only be a consequence of a more serious underlying pathology but, irrespective of its pathophysiology, an arrhythmia may pose a serious risk or a difficult medical problem. Tachyarrhythmias must therefore be diagnosed and treated with great care and expertise.

For too long the cardiologist and the arrhythmologist/electrophysiologist have guarded their professional skills as secrets. In the past, the physician used the electrocardiogram and the electrophysiological study to establish accurate diagnoses, but the therapeutic consequences of these erudite diagnoses were negligible until the advent of electrophysiological surgery. Now the introduction of techniques of catheter ablation have catapulted cardiac electrophysiology into the medical headlines.

The mechanism of a cardiac arrhythmia is fundamentally important if therapy can be directed specifically toward that mechanism. Without knowledge of the target, the therapy cannot be aimed in the right direction. Some of our more successful therapies are "blunderbuss" treatments, such as amiodarone and the implantable cardioverter defibrillator. Irrespective of the cause of the arrhythmia, one of the many actions of amiodarone may well solve or suppress the problem. The cause of ventricular fibrillation is largely irrelevant to the corrective action

v

taken by the implanted defibrillator. However, knowing, for example, that conduction through the right bundle branch is a critical component of bundle branch reentrant tachycardia, identifies an easy target for ablation therapy. Similarly, knowledge about the cellular mechanisms responsible for the long QT syndrome suggests obvious and specific antiarrhythmic medical and surgical approaches to the treatment. This specific approach to therapy, suggested recently in the *Sicilian Gambit,* must sometimes be at arm's length—applying assumptions from tissue or animal models to the human clinical situation. On the other hand, the much more detailed deductions that can now be drawn from the surface electrocardiogram and from intracardiac electrophysiological recordings now allow the electrophysiologist to make measurements and experiments directly on the culprit arrhythmia. The effect of therapeutic interventions may then be easily reassessed and further therapeutic measures can be instituted until all is well.

The aim of this series of monographs, devoted to cardiac arrhythmology, is to update the physician and cardiologist and all of those responsible for caring for patients with cardiac arrhythmias about the spectacular developments in diagnostic and interventional cardiac electrophysiology. Hardly an arrhythmia fails to yield to the skills of the modern arrhythmologist. He no longer needs secrets; his successes are plain for all to see.

A. John Camm, M.D., Series Editor
Chairman of Medicine and Chief
Department of Cardiological Sciences
St. George's Hospital Medical School
London University
London United Kingdom

Preface

Ventricular tachyarrhythmias cause the majority of sudden cardiac deaths. Many victims of out-of hospital cardiac arrest are now successfully resuscitated in the community by paramedic rescue teams. The potential to suffer from life-threatening arrhythmias has been identified in many groups of patients. The treatment of those rescued from sudden arrhythmic death or of those known to be at some risk from such arrhythmias cannot be effectively or cheaply accomplished with antiarrhythmic drugs. However, although we still await conclusive clinical trial confirmation, the use of an implantable cardioverter-defibrillator (ICD) does seem efficacious in these patients. This therapy is expensive, at least initially, and extensive use of the technology cannot be afforded by many, if not most, health care systems.

Not every patient in a high-risk group of patients will suffer a fatal ventricular arrhythmia; in some instances, only a minority will do so. Not all ventricular tachyarrhythmias are likely to kill patients. Identification as a potential victim of sudden death is often psychologically debilitating and some therapies are themselves hazardous; for example, the use of drugs that may be pro-arrhythmic rather than antiarrhythmic. Treatment with the ICD may be expensive, possibly complicated (operative mortality, infections, displacements, hematomas, erosions, etc.), often socially difficult (loss of driving privileges, etc.), and occasionally difficult to tolerate. There-fore, accurate identification of those at risk is essential.

Inspection of trials of treatment of conventionally identified "high-risk" patients allows the mortality of placebo groups or, in the case of ICD treated patients, the discharge rate of the device to be evaluated. Such studies demonstrate that our ability to predict the occurrence of ventricular tachyarrhythmias is at best modest. It is un-acceptable to "ration" health care, but on the other hand, it is not possible to afford indiscriminate provision of es-sentially unnecessary health care; neither is this sensible. It is, therefore, important to improve the accuracy of our diagnostic techniques, a major component of which is the assessment of prognosis. We must know which patient needs specific treatments. Risk stratification is an impor-tant technique that must be applied to patients who may, but might not, be "at risk" of suffering from fatal ventric-ular tachyarrhythmias.

Our prognostication skills are not yet good enough; this state of affairs must be improved. In this volume of the Clinical Approaches to Tachyarrhythmias Series, Mark Anderson reviews the present state of our know-ledge.

A. John Camm, M.D.
Series Editor

Contents

Introduction: Epidemiology of Ventricular Tachyarrhythmias

For over a century, it has been recognized that ventricular tachyarrhythmias may be associated with an adverse prognosis. In 1889, John McWilliam,[1] while reviewing the subject of sudden death, wrote that ". . . . it is very probable that in many of these cases the fatal issue is determined or ensured by the occurrence of fibrillar contraction in the ventricles."

Sudden death is now recognized as a common mode of death in the Western world with approximately 400,000 such deaths per annum in the United States.[2,3] The majority of such sudden deaths appears to be due to cardiac disease and, particularly, coronary artery disease. Evidence from community studies such as the Wandsworth study[4] suggests that ischemic heart disease is responsible for about 65% of sudden deaths in men and 40% in women. In the same study, nonischemic cardiac disease was responsible for 6% of deaths in men and 12% in women. Although there has been some debate over the precise definition of what constitutes a sudden cardiac death,[5] data from a number of studies suggest that between 70% and 90% of such deaths are arrhythmic in origin.[6,7]

1

Table 1

Noncoronary Artery Disease Associated with Ventricular Tachyarrhythmias

Dilated cardiomyopathy
Hypertrophic cardiomyopathy
Pregnancy
Sarcoidosis
Chagas' disease
Long QT syndrome
Coronary artery spasm
Wolff-Parkinson-White syndrome
Mitral valve prolapse
Right ventricular dysplasia
Normal heart

Estimation of the proportion of sudden cardiac deaths, where there is evidence suggestive of acute myocardial infarction, varies from 35% to 70%.[8-12] Of all sudden cardiac deaths, only 40% occur in patients with a prior history of cardiac disease,[13] and only a small proportion of these patients will have a prior history of ventricular arrhythmia. Nonetheless, because of the increasing development of out-of-hospital resuscitation,[14,15] more patients who would die a sudden cardiac death survive to leave the hospital, and there has been considerable interest in the identification of patients at high risk of recurrent life-threatening arrhythmias.

Not all patients with ventricular tachyarrhythmias present with cardiac arrest. Symptomatic sustained ventricular tachycardia (VT), symptomatic nonsustained VT (NSVT), and asymptomatic NSVT detected by Holter monitoring constitute the remainder. It is surprising, in view of their relative frequency, that there are no large-scale studies of the annual incidence of ventricular arrhythmias that do not result in cardiac arrest. Sustained VT usually results in symptoms that lead the patient to seek medical attention and treatment. Therefore, the prevalence of sustained VT is low. While numerous studies have documented a high incidence of ventricular extrasystoles during Holter monitoring in normal people,[16] NSVT can be found in only 0.5% or less of the population.[17]

Over 90% of patients presenting with ventricular tachyarrhythmias have coronary artery disease, but a variety of etiologies are found in the remainder (Table 1).

Why Risk Assessment?

Risk assessment in such patients serves a number of purposes. It enables both the identification of patients who may benefit from specific antiarrhythmic therapies such as drugs, surgery, or the implantable cardioverter-defibrillator (ICD) and the evaluation of the risk-benefit and cost-benefit relationships of using these treatments. Because of the potential for sudden incapacitation associated with ventricular tachyarrhythmias, risk assessment also enables patients to be given rational advice concerning incapacitation-sensitive activities such as driving. Finally, information from risk assessment is important to patients who wish to have some idea of their long-term prognosis.

Increasing emphasis on the use of large-scale randomized clinical trials of pharmaceutical and interventional therapies has greatly facilitated the development of the science of risk assessment by focusing on the natural history of cardiac disease in the untreated and treated states. Risk assessment has a role in selecting the most appropriate therapy for the individual patient, but increasingly is being applied as a tool for social and medical planning.

Risk Assessment Techniques

A wide range of techniques are available to assist in the process of risk assessment. These techniques and the potentially useful data derived from them are summarized in Table 2.

Most work on risk assessment has been conducted in patients with coronary artery disease and this area is considered first. The limited data on risk assessment in patients with ventricular tachyarrhythmias due to other etiologies are considered in the latter part of this book.

Table 2

Techniques for Risk Assessment of Patients Presenting with Ventricular Tachyarrhythmias

Technique	Derived Information	Invasive
Clinical history and examination	Age, heart failure, previous heart disease	
Electrocardiogram	Presenting arrhythmia	
	Presence of old infarction	
Echocardiogram	Ejection fraction	
Nuclear angiogram	Ejection fraction	
Holter tape	Ventricular premature beats	
	Nonsustained ventricular tachycardia	
	Heart rate variability	
Signal-averaged electrocardiogram	Late potentials	
Exercise testing	Excercise-induced arrhythmia, ischemia	
Coronary angiography	Coronary anatomy	X
	Ejection fraction	
Electrophysiological study	Inducibility of arrhythmias	X

Risk Assessment of Ventricular Tachyarrhythmias in Patients with Coronary Artery Disease

Early Postinfarction Ventricular Fibrillation

Ventricular fibrillation (VF) occurring within 48 hours of acute myocardial infarction is not an indicator of risk for subsequent ventricular tachyarrhythmias and any slight adverse impact on survival is confined to the in-hospital phase of recovery.[18,19] Risk assessment in patients with an episode of VF in the first 48 hours should follow the same course as for patients who do not suffer an arrhythmia. Risk assessment in patients following uncomplicated myocardial infarction has been extensively considered elsewhere and will not be reviewed further in this book. Ventricular arrhythmias occurring after 48 hours are associated with extensive infarction, poorer left ventricular function, and higher mortality (Fig. 1).[20,21] Arrhythmias occurring in the first few weeks following infarction may be associated with a higher mortality than those occurring later.

Sustained Ventricular Tachyarrhythmias in Patients with Coronary Artery Disease Occurring in the Absence of Acute Myocardial Infarction

There has been intense interest in the risk stratification of myocardial infarction survivors[22-24] to identify those patients who will suffer a late arrhythmic event. Despite the use of combinations of screening tests, the construction of a risk stratification strategy of sufficient sensitivity and specificity to make the application of

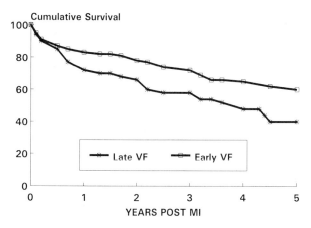

Figure 1. Prognosis of patients developing VF early (<48 hours) or late (≥48 hours) after myocardial infarction. Reproduced with permission from Jensen GV, Torp-Pedersen C, Kober L, Steensgaard-Hansen F, Rasmussen YH, Berning J, et al. Prognosis of late versus early ventricular fibrillation in acute myocardial infarction. Am J Cardiol 1990;66:10-15.

prophylactic antiarrhythmic therapies to infarct survivors has been difficult. However, patients with coronary artery disease, with or without prior myocardial infarction, who present with a ventricular tachyarrhythmia have identified themselves as being at high risk. Early studies have shown that cardiac arrest survivors may have a recurrence rate as high as 30% at one year and 45% at two years.[25-27]

Clinical Variables: The use of clinical variables alone may enable the identification of patients at high risk of further arrhythmia. The Dutch Ventricular Tachycardia

Table 3

Clinical Variables in Patients with Ventricular Tachyarrhythmias and Coronary Artery Disease Associated with Subsequent Total Mortality

Variable	Risk Ratio (RR)	95% CI of RR	P Value
First VT/VF <6 Weeks after MI			
Age >70 years	4.5	2.6–7.7	0.00001
Cardiac arrest	1.7	1.0–2.8	0.0025
Killip Class III or IV	3.5	1.5–4.4	0.0031
Anterior MI	2.2	1.2–3.9	0.0158
Multiple previous MIs	1.6	0.9–2.7	0.1057
First VT/VF >6 Weeks after MI			
Q-wave MI	2.1	0.8–5.9	0.0734
Cardiac arrest	1.7	1.1–2.9	0.0455
Killip Class III or IV	1.7	0.8–3.4	0.1861
Multiple previous MIs	1.4	0.8–2.4	0.2559

MI: Myocardial infarction
Reproduced with permission from Willems AR, Tijssen JGP, van Cappelle FJL, Kingma JH, Hauer RN, Vermeulen FE, et al. Determinants of prognosis in symptomatic ventricular tachycardia or ventricular fibrillation late after myocardial infarction. J Am Coll Cardiol 1990; 16:521–530.

Study Group of the Interuniversity Institute of the Netherlands has published an analysis of clinical factors associated with subsequent mortality in 390 patients presenting with sustained symptomatic VT or VF occurring more than 48 hours after myocardial infarction.[28] The Cox proportional hazards model was used to identify clinical characteristics that were independent predictors of subsequent total mortality. The results of this analysis are summarized in Table 3 and show that early ventricular arrhythmia (>48 hours and <6 weeks postinfarction), age

>70 years, presentation with cardiac arrest, Killip Class III or IV heart failure, and prior anterior myocardial infarction are significantly associated with subsequent mortality. For arrhythmias occurring after six weeks, only presentation with cardiac arrest emerged as a significant factor.

Invasive Electrophysiological Assessment and the Role of Ejection Fraction: Since the development of programmed ventricular stimulation in the mid-1970s by Josephson and colleagues,[29] this technique has become widely established as a means of risk assessment for patients who have presented with a sustained ventricular tachyarrhythmia. Its ability to allow induction of the clinically relevant arrhythmia and the relative ease with which it may be repeated to allow assessment of the impact of antiarrhythmic drug therapy are among the reasons for its widespread use. In patients presenting with sustained VT, the presence of inducible sustained monomorphic VT (SMVT) is a powerful univariate predictor with a relative risk for total mortality of 4.20 and a relative risk of 4.35 for arrhythmia recurrence.[30] Wilber and colleagues[31] have shown that failure to suppress inducible VT in patients presenting with cardiac arrest is similarly associated with a much higher rate of recurrent cardiac arrest (Fig. 2), a finding replicated by many other studies.[32,33]

Protocols: The comparability of data from different studies is restricted by the use of differing stimulation protocols for the electrophysiological study (EPS). The opti-

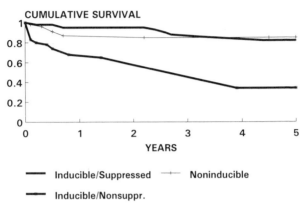

Figure 2. Cumulative survival in patients surviving a cardiac arrest stratified by EPS. Inducible/Suppressed: inducible arrhythmia with suppression by antiarrhythmic drug therapy; Inducible/Nonsuppr.: inducible arrhythmia not suppressed by antiarrhythmic drug therapy. Reproduced with permission from Wilber DJ, Garan H, Finkelstein D, Kelly E, Newell J, McGovern B, et al. Out-of-hospital cardiac arrest. Use of electrophysiological testing in the prediction of long-term survival. N Engl J Med 1988;318:19-24.

mum yield of tachycardia induction in patients presenting with ventricular tachyarrhythmias has been shown to be achieved using a 400 millisecond drive cycle with up to four extra stimuli (Fig. 3).[34] However, increasing the number of extrastimuli used is known to reduce the specificity and repeatability of testing.[35,36] Results of repeat EPSs separated by a period of days show kappa (κ) values of 0.5 to 0.6 for noninducibility or inducibility of sustained VT, indicating only a moderate degree of reproducibility.[37] Repeat studies performed within a few minutes of each other show better reproducibility.[38]

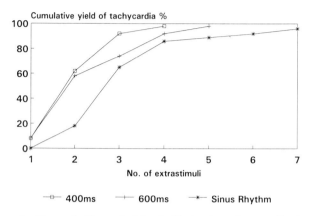

Figure 3. Cumulative yield of clinical tachycardia induction at EPS versus drive cycle and number of extrastimuli. Reproduced with permission from Ho DSW, Cooper MJ, Richards DAB, Uther JB, Yip ASB, Ross DL. Comparison of number of extrastimuli versus change in basic cycle length for induction of ventricular tachycardia by programmed ventricular stimulation. J Am Coll Cardiol 1993;22:1711-1717.

End Points: The occurrence of SMVT is accepted by all as an indication of a positive EPS. Nonsustained or polymorphic VT induction are less satisfactory end points[37,39] because of their poor reproducibility. Similarly, inducible VF has not been shown to be a useful marker for risk assessment.[40] Basic guidelines for stimulation protocols during EPSs have been defined by the North American Society of Pacing and Electrophysiology.[41] The type of arrhythmia induced varies depending on the clinical presentation (Fig. 4).[42] In more than 90% of patients pre-

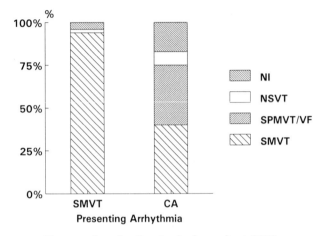

Figure 4. Type of arrhythmia induced at EPS versus arrhythmia at clinical presentation. NI: noninducible; NSVT: nonsustained VT; SPMVT/VF: sustained polymorphic VT/VF; SMVT: sustained monomorphic VT; CA: cardiac arrest. Reproduced with permission from Josephson ME. Recurrent ventricular tachycardia. In Clinical Cardiac Electrophysiology: Techniques and Interpretations. Philadelphia: Lea & Fabiger, 1993.

senting with SMVT, an SMVT can be induced at EPS. In cardiac arrest survivors, this figure falls to 40%. In many studies, these two types of patients have been present in varying proportions and this accounts for the variability of the findings and reproducibility of EPSs in different reports.

Risk Assessment for Antiarrhythmic Drug Therapy: The finding of an antiarrhythmic drug that suppresses the in-

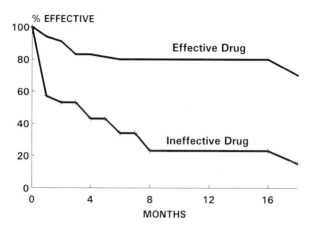

Figure 5. Incidence of arrhythmia recurrence is significantly reduced ($P<0.001$) in patients (n = 39) with a prediction of antiarrhythmic drug efficacy versus those (n = 17) in whom no effective drug is found. Reproduced with permission from Mason JW, Winkle RA. Accuracy of the ventricular tachycardia-induction study for predicting long-term efficacy and inefficacy of antiarrhythmic drugs. New Engl J Med 1980;303:1073-1077.

duction of previously inducible VT is associated with a reduced incidence of arrhythmia recurrence from 67% to 20% at six months (Fig. 5).[43] However, successful suppression of an inducible arrhythmia by an antiarrhythmic drug is not an absolute phenomenon as repeated attempts at induction using the same protocol may eventually succeed in inducing the ventricular arrhythmia in over 60% of patients.[44,45] This reflects the essentially probabilistic nature of the EPS. Slowing of the induced tachycardia without complete abolition has also been reported to be associated with a reduction in mortality, although not in

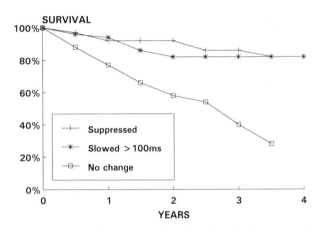

Figure 6. Impact of slowing of arrhythmia by antiarrhythmic drugs on total survival. Suppressed: total suppression by drugs of arrhythmia inducibility; Slowed >100 ms: slowing of inducible tachycardia by at least 100 ms cycle length; No change: tachycardia remains inducible with less than 100 ms change in cycle length. Reproduced with permission from Waller TJ, Kay HR, Spielman SR, Kutalek SP, Greenspan AM, Horowitz LN. Reduction in sudden death and total mortality by antiarrhythmic therapy evaluated by electrophysiologic drug testing: Criteria of efficacy in patients with sustained ventricular tachyarrhythmia. J Am Coll Cardiol 1987;10:83-89.

arrhythmia recurrence rate (Fig. 6).[46] A successful response to a single antiarrhythmic agent is associated with a successful response to other agents.[47] Kavanagh and coworkers[48] have shown that the likelihood of finding an effective suppressive antiarrhythmic drug therapy falls from 23% at the first trials to 9% at the second and third trials and to 5% at the fourth trial (Fig. 7). Additionally, whereas drugs identified in the first three trials seem to

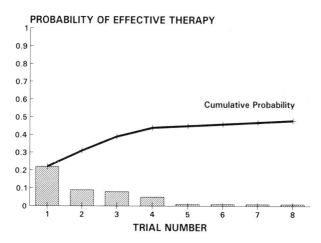

Figure 7. Probability of a prediction of antiarrhythmic drug efficacy at successive drug trials. There is a steady fall in the likelihood of finding a drug predicted to be effective at successive studies. Reproduced with permission from Kavanagh KM, Wyse G, Duff HJ, Gillis AM, Sheldon RS, Mitchell LB. Drug therapy for ventricular tachyarrhythmias: How many electropharmacological trials are appropriate. J Am Coll Cardiol 1991;17:391-396.

have a roughly similar level of efficacy in the long term, an apparently effective drug identified after more than three previous drug trial failures is less likely to be effective in the long term (Fig. 8). Particular questions have been raised concerning the usefulness of EP testing to assess the response to amiodarone therapy.[49] Effective suppression of arrhythmia by amiodarone has been reported to reduce the actuarial probability of arrhythmia recurrence at 24 months from 48% to 3%, even in patients who had previously failed an average of four antiarrhythmic drug trials.[50] In this study, as in many others, ejection fraction was significantly higher in the group without ar-

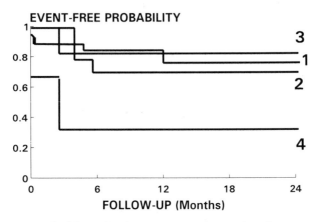

Figure 8. Likelihood of remaining free of arrhythmia re-currence when treated with an antiarrhythmic drug pre-dicted to be effective at EPS at the first (1), second (2), third (3), or fourth (4) drug trial. An antiarrhythmic drug iden-tified as suppressive after multiple previous trials may be less effective than expected. Reproduced with permission from Kavanagh KM, Wyse G, Duff HJ, Gillis AM, Sheldon RS, Mitchell LB. Drug therapy for ventricular tachy-arrhythmias: How many electropharmacological trials are appropriate. J Am Coll Cardiol 1991;17:391-396.

rhythmia recurrence. The Cardiac Arrest in Seattle: Con-ventional Versus Amiodarone Drug Evaluation (CAS-CADE) study[51] compared total survival and survival free of recurrent ventricular tachyarrhythmias in cardiac ar-rest survivors resuscitated from VF randomized to con-ventional electrophysiology-guided or Holter-guided drug therapy or blind amiodarone therapy. The survival results are summarized in Figure 9 and suggest that blind amiodarone therapy may be more efficacious than con-ventional drug therapy guided by either means.

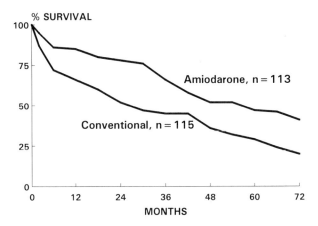

Figure 9. Survival free of cardiac death and sustained arrhythmia in cardiac arrest patients randomized to conventional EP-guided antiarrhythmic drug therapy versus amiodarone. Data from the Cascade Investigators.[51]

Left Ventricular Ejection Fraction: Implications for Risk Stratification by Electrophysiological Study: Reduced left ventricular ejection fraction is a powerful predictor of mortality after myocardial infarction.[52,53] In patients presenting with cardiac arrest or SMVT, it is strongly associated with the likelihood of recurrence[30,31] (Fig. 10), and this observation has been confirmed by experience with implantable defibrillators where patients with lower ejection fractions are more likely to receive a device therapy and do so sooner.[54,55] In the study by Wilber et al,[31] the result of the EP testing added additional predictive information to that derived from ejection fraction alone. However, in this study, the ejection fraction was treated as a dichotomized variable (ejection fraction [EF] >30% or <30%). This results in the loss of much of the informa-

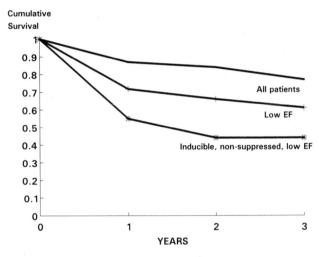

Figure 10. Survival free of further cardiac arrest in cardiac arrest survivors with a left ventricular ejection fraction of ≤30% (Low EF) and those with an inducible arrhythmia, not suppressed by antiarrhythmic drug therapy in addition to Low EF (Inducible, non-suppressed, low EF). Reproduced with permission from Wilber DJ, Garan H, Finkelstein D, Kelly E, Newell J, McGovern B, et al. Out-of-hospital cardiac arrest. Use of electrophysiological testing in the prediction of long-term survival. N Engl J Med 1988;318:19-24.

tion obtained by measurement of ejection fraction. Those studies in which ejection fraction has been treated as a continuous variable[30] suggest that left ventricular function is the dominant factor determining outcome with marginal additional information being obtained from the EPS. In a study of 47 patients at St. George's Hospital, London, who received an implantable defibrillator and who were followed for an average of 17.05 months, six variables showed a statistically significant association with appropriate ICD therapy delivery (which equates to arrhythmia recurrence) by univariate analysis. These were left ventricular ejection fraction, left ventricular end-diastolic diameter, heart diameter on posteroanterior chest x-ray, inducibility of ventricular arrhythmia at EPS, presentation with sustained VT, and continued antiarrhythmic drug therapy. Cox's proportional hazard model was used to examine these variables and to quantify the proportional hazard of therapy delivery associated with each percentage point fall in ejection fraction. Of the six variables, the Cox model selected left ventricular ejection fraction as the single variable best predicting the occurrence of appropriate therapy delivery. The relative risk (per 1% fall in ejection fraction) was 1.04 (χ-squared 11.69). Inclusion of any of the other variables (including inducibility of arrhythmia at EPS) failed to improve the "fit" of the model. Figure 11 shows the difference in survival free of appropriate ICD therapy (= arrhythmia recurrence) observed between inducible and noninducible patients, and the hypothetical difference in survival when the effect of ejection fraction differences between the groups are removed.

Thus, while inducibility at EPS may be a useful means of assessing response to antiarrhythmic drug therapy, it provides little additional information over and above that from the ejection fraction for primary risk assessment.

Holter Recording: Holter recording has been advocated as an alternative method for risk assessment in patients presenting with ventricular tachyarrhythmias. A number of nonrandomized studies has been conducted comparing outcome after evaluation of antiarrhythmic drug regimens by Holter monitoring or EPS.[56,57] However, only two stud-

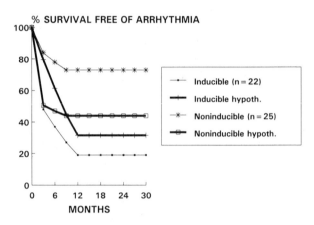

Figure 11. The impact of using ejection fraction as a clinical variable on the information derived from EPS. If ejection fraction is ignored, inducibility at EPS appears to be a discriminator of survival free of arrhythmia. When the impact of ejection fraction is allowed for (Inducible hypoth. and Noninducible hypoth.), most of the discriminant power is eroded. Unpublished data on 47 patients from the St. George's Hospital, London, implantable defibrillator data base.

ies have randomized patients to the two approaches. Mitchell and colleagues[58] conducted a small study in 57 patients randomly assigned to noninvasive or invasive risk assessment. The criteria of efficacy for the Holter recording group was suppression of more than 80% of isolated premature ventricular beats, more than 90% of couplets, and 100% of triplets and longer repetitive forms. Predicted effective drug therapy was identified in all 29 patients randomized to the noninvasive group and in 54% of the 28 patients randomized to the invasive approach.

Patients in this group in whom no predicted therapy could be identified were treated with empiric amiodarone therapy. At the end of 24 months, actuarial likelihood of remaining arrhythmia recurrence free was 0.50 ± 0.10 in the noninvasive group and 0.80 ± 0.08 in the invasive group. The small size of this study made it impossible to draw any conclusions about overall mortality. The much larger Electrophysiologic Study Versus Electrocardiographic Monitoring (ESVEM) trial[59] randomized 486 patients to the two therapeutic approaches. The criteria for efficacy in the Holter group was suppression of 70% of all ventricular premature contractions (VPCs), 80% of pairs, 90% of runs of <15 beats of VT, and 100% of longer runs. In the EPS group, the definition of efficacy was suppression of VT lasting more than 15 beats. Drug efficacy was predicted in 77% of the Holter group and 45% in the EPS group. Time taken to identify an effective therapy was similar in both groups. Long-term follow-up over six years showed no significant difference in the recurrence rate of arrhythmia (Figure 12) or mortality in the two groups in whom a prediction of treatment efficacy was obtained.[60]

Ventricular Premature Contractions: The presence of VPCs and particularly of complex multimorphic forms in survivors of myocardial infarction is known to be associated with an increased risk of sudden cardiac death,[61,62] but difficulties with the Lown classification of multimorphic forms[63] and the strong interrelationship between ventricular ectopics and left ventricular function[64] limit their usefulness. No studies have examined the relationship between the occurrence of VPCs and the incidence of recurrent arrhythmias in patients presenting with ventricular arrhythmias.

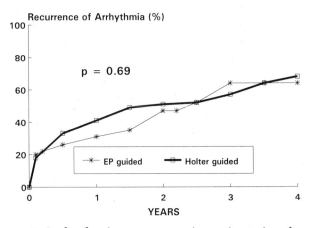

Figure 12. Arrhythmia recurrence in patients in whom antiarrhythmic drug efficacy has been predicted by invasive EPS (EP guided) or by Holter monitoring (Holter guided). Data from Mason JW for the Electrophysiologic Study versus Electrocardiographic Monitoring Investigators study.[60]

Heart Rate Variability: Like the VPC count, heart rate variability (HRV) has been widely used as a risk stratification tool after myocardial infarction,[65,66] where it may be even more powerful than assessment of the ejection fraction. About 80% of patients with coronary artery disease and inducible VT have abnormal HRV by spectral analysis.[67] Reductions in total power of HRV are known to occur in the hour prior to the occurrence of VT,[68] but not prior to the occurrence of VF.[69] Whether HRV is a useful tool for risk stratification in patients who have suffered a cardiac arrest or sustained VT is not yet clear.

Signal-Averaged Electrocardiogram: A positive signal-averaged electrocardiogram (ECG) is known to be associated with a propensity to ventricular tachyarrhythmias in postmyocardial infarction patients.[70,71] In combination with HRV, it may provide a powerful index of arrhythmia risk.[65,72] However, its value in risk stratification of patients who have already sustained a spontaneous ventricular tachyarrhythmia remains to be shown. Dolack and colleagues[73] were unable to demonstrate any association between the presence of inducible VT and a positive signal-averaged ECG in 25 patients with recurrent sustained VT and 46 survivors of out-of-hospital VF, and it does not appear to predict delivery of appropriate implantable defibrillator therapies.[74]

Exercise Testing: The occurrence of ventricular arrhythmias on exercise has not been shown to be a useful independent predictor of cardiac events or mortality in patients with coronary artery disease.[75,76] Serious exercise-induced arrhythmias are relatively uncommon in patients with coronary artery disease and, when associated with ischemia, there is good evidence that coronary artery bypass grafting alleviates both the ischemia and the arrhythmia.[77] The reproducibility of exercise-induced VT in patients presenting with VT or VF is low with kappa (κ) values of <0.2.[78] Although testing for exercise-induced arrhythmias was included as part of the noninvasive protocol in the ESVEM study only, the study was not formally designed to assess the efficacy of exercise testing as a risk assessment technique. In the opinion of the investigators, "exercise testing as we applied it does not add sufficient information to Holter Monitoring to justify its use as a means to validate efficacy predictions by Holter Monitoring."[59]

Coronary Angiography: To establish a cardiac diagnosis, patients presenting with sustained VT or cardiac arrest usually undergo coronary arteriography. Additionally, ischemia may have a role to play in the etiology of some episodes of arrhythmia. Around one third of patients with an inducible arrhythmia prior to coronary artery bypass grafting are rendered noninducible subsequently.[79] No controlled study has examined the relationship between the extent of coronary disease and recurrence rate of arrhythmias. Since coronary disease tends to be aggressively treated in patients presenting with ventricular tachyarrhythmias, it would be difficult to carry out such a trial.

Combinations of Risk Assessment Techniques: The potential power of combining risk assessment techniques has been extensively explored in postmyocardial infarction patients,[65,72] but has yet to be applied in the risk assessment of patients presenting with ventricular tachyarrhythmias.

Nonsustained Ventricular Tachycardia in Patients with Coronary Artery Disease

Most investigators have defined NSVT as $\geq$3 beats of hemodynamically stable VT at a rate of >120 beats/minute terminating spontaneously in <30 seconds. Nonsustained VT is known to be associated with increased sudden and nonsudden cardiac mortality following myocardial infarction.[80-82] As with sustained VT, a wide variety of risk assessment techniques has been applied to patients with NSVT. Their primary aim has been less to predict the risk of further episodes of NSVT and more to predict the risk of sustained VT or VF. A limitation of all studies of NSVT is that the incidence is highly dependent on the frequency of Holter recording and may alter spontaneously over time.[83]

Ejection Fraction: As in patients with sustained ventricular tachyarrhythmias, left ventricular ejection fraction is a powerful predictor of outcome in patients with NSVT.[84-86] In the study of Kowey et al,[86] recurrent arrhythmia rates were 7% in the normal group (EF >50%), 22% in the mildly impaired group (EF 35% to 50%), and 71% in the moderately impaired group (EF <35%).

Invasive Electrophysiological Studies: The role of EPSs in risk assessment of patients with NSVT remains controversial. A large number of noncontrolled studies has suggested that EPSs can identify patients at higher risk of recurrent ventricular arrhythmias (Fig. 13).[87-89] Kowey and colleagues[90] conducted a meta-analysis of 12 papers on this topic published since 1986. A sustained ventricular tachyarrhythmia could be induced in 302 (33%) of the 926 patients included in these studies. Over a mean 19.4 month follow-up, 18% of inducible patients suffered an arrhythmic event compared with 7% of noninducible patients. Sensitivity of inducible arrhythmia for subsequent arrhythmic event was 54%, specificity 70%, positive predictive accuracy 18%, and negative predictive accuracy 93%. This suggests that noninducibility at EPS may be a useful way of identifying patients at low risk of subsequent arrhythmia, but the possible confounding effects of ejection fraction were not considered by this study. In a retrospective study of 205 patients conducted by the Philadelphia Arrhythmia Group, programmed stimula-

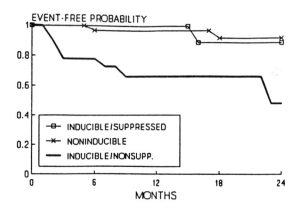

Figure 13. Freedom from arrhythmic event in patients presenting with NSVT predicted by EPS. INDUCIBLE/SUPPRESSED: inducible arrhythmia with suppression by antiarrhythmic drug therapy; INDUCIBLE/NONSUPP.: inducible arrhythmia not suppressed by antiarrhythmic drug therapy. Reproduced with permission from Wilber DJ, Olshansky B, Moran JF, Scanlon PJ. Electrophysiological testing and nonsustained ventricular tachycardia. Circulation 1990;82:350-358. Copyright 1990 American Heart Association.

tion did not have independent predictive value of arrhythmia recurrence, once the confounding effect of ejection fraction had been removed.[86] Realistically, only a randomized controlled trial will be able to answer whether EPSs are of use in the risk assessment of patients with NSVT. Two such trials are currently in progress, both recruiting patients with ejection fractions below 40% (Fig. 14). The Multicenter Unsustained Tachycardia Trial (MUSTT) compares EP-guided drug therapy with placebo for patients with inducible arrhythmia.[91] In the EP-guided group, patients who remain inducible despite drug ther-

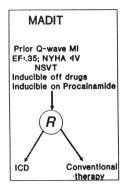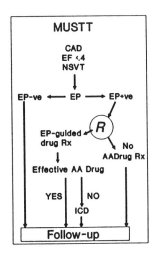

Figure 14. The design of the MUSTT[91] and MADIT[92] trials designed to assess risk assessment of patients with NSVT. MI: myocardial infarction; NYHA<IV: not in New York Heart Association Grade IV; CAD: coronary artery disease; EF: ejection fraction; NSVT: nonsustained VT; EP: electrophysiological study; EP + ve: inducible sustained ventricular arrhythmias at EPS; EP − ve: no sustained ventricular arrhythmias at EPS; F/U: follow-up; R: randomization; AA Drug: antiarrhythmic drug; ICD: implantable cardioverter-defibrillator.

apy receive an ICD. Patients who are not inducible are not part of the study, but their outcome is followed up and this trial will provide information on the impact of EPSs and the effect of EP-guided therapy on the outcome in patients with NSVT. The Multicenter Automatic Defibrillator Implantation Trial (MADIT)[92] recruits patients with NSVT who have inducible arrhythmias at baseline EPS that remain inducible on procainamide. These patients are randomized to ICD or "conventional" EP-guided drug therapy to test the hypothesis that the ICD is superior to conventional therapy (decided by the recruiting physician). Both studies will provide information on the natural history of arrhythmias in patients with NSVT.

Holter Monitoring: Although this is useful for documenting the recurrence of asymptomatic episodes of NSVT, it has not been shown to be useful in risk assessment of NSVT patients.

Heart Rate Variability: There have been no formal studies of the usefulness of HRV in risk assessment of NSVT patients.

Signal-Averaged Electrocardiogram: The signal-averaged ECG appears to be a useful screening test for inducibility of VT during EPS in patients with NSVT[93,94] with an excellent negative predictive value. It may therefore be useful in identifying patients who do not need referral for EPS. Its role as an independent risk assessment tool in patients with NSVT has not been evaluated.

Ventricular Tachyarrhythmias in Noncoronary Artery Disease Patients

A wide range of noncoronary cardiac disease is associated with the occurrence of ventricular tachyarrhythmias (Table 2).

Normal Heart

Ventricular tachycardia can occur in the absence of any recognized cardiac disease, although persistent investigation in patients without overt disease may identify subtle abnormalities such as right ventricular dysplasia[95] or possible autonomic dysfunction.[96] Four different patterns of idiopathic VT have been described based on the bundle branch block pattern and frontal QRS axis.[97] These are summarized in Table 4. The right bundle branch block right axis (RBBBRA) group appears to have a distinct mechanism from the other groups involving bundle branch reentry. This type of tachycardia is responsive to verapamil,[98] but rarely occurs during exercise. The re-

Table 4

Occurrence of Different Electrocardiographic Patterns in 47 Patients with "Normal Heart" Ventricular Tachycardia

Bundle Branch Pattern	Frontal QRS axis	N (%)	Group
RBBB	Left or superior	9 (19)	RBBBLA
RBBB	Normal or right axis	9 (19)	RBBBRA
LBBB	Left or superior	5 (11)	LBBBLA
LBBB	Normal or right	24 (51)	LBBBRA

RBBB: right bundle branch block; RBBBLA: right bundle branch block left axis; RBBBRA: right bundle branch block right axis; LBBB: left bundle branch block; LBBBLA: left bundle branch block left axis; LBBBRA: left bundle branch block right axis. Reproduced with permission from Mont L, Seixas T, Brugada P, Brugada J, Simonis F, Kriek E, et al. The electrocardiographic, clinical, and electrophysiologic spectrum of idiopathic monomorphic ventricular tachycardia. Am Heart J 1992; 124:746–753.

maining patterns of normal heart VT have a high incidence (40% to 75%) of induction during exercise testing, suggesting a role for catecholamines and the autonomic nervous system. No randomized prospective study of patients with normal heart VT has been published, but in the study by Lemery and colleagues,[99] of the 47 patients with normal heart VT, there was no mortality from sudden cardiac death or arrhythmias after a mean follow-up of 96 months, although there are isolated reports of sudden death.[100] There is a significant arrhythmia recurrence rate in these patients despite medical therapy (Fig. 15), but radiofre-

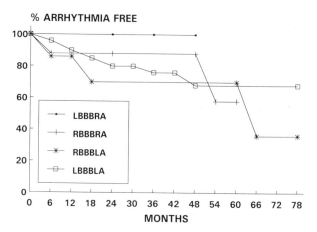

Figure 15. Recurrence rate of VT for different patterns of normal heart VT. RBBBRA: right bundle branch block right axis; RBBBLA: right bundle branch block left axis; LBBBRA: left bundle branch block right axis; LBBBLA: left bundle branch block left axis. Reproduced with permission from Mont L, Seixas T, Brugada P, Brugada J, Simonis F, Kriek E, et al. The electrocardiographic, clinical, and electrophysiologic spectrum of idiopathic monomorphic ventricular tachycardia. Am Heart J 1992;124:746-753.

quency ablation has been reported to be a successful therapy in all of these patients.[101] No prospective evaluation of risk assessment techniques has been described in normal heart VT patients. The incidence of late potentials in these patients is much lower than in patients with ischemic heart disease and VT,[102] and while spectral HRV is significantly lower in sudden cardiac death survivors with normal hearts than in controls,[103] the use of this parameter to identify high-risk patients has not been evaluated. Currently, therefore, no specific advice on risk assessment of these patients can be provided.

The occurrence of VT during pregnancy has been widely reported, although its frequency is unknown. It is unclear whether these patients are simply part of the spectrum of normal heart VT or represent a true diagnostic category. Most reports suggest a good outcome for these patients,[104] and no risk assessment techniques have been systematically applied.

Hypertrophic Cardiomyopathy

Cardiac Arrest: The association of hypertrophic cardiomyopathy (HOCM) with sudden cardiac death is well recognized with an annual mortality in adults from this cause of 2% to 3%.[105] The precise mechanism of sudden cardiac death in HOCM patients remains conjectural, but in the one published case of Holter monitoring during death, the terminal event was initiated by VPCs followed by rapid polymorphic VT.[106] Resuscitated survivors of sudden cardiac death remain a management problem. In their study of 33 resuscitated survivors of cardiac arrest in HOCM patients, Cecchi and colleagues[107] reported a recurrent cardiac arrest rate of 35% at five years (Fig. 16). This experience predates the widespread availability of

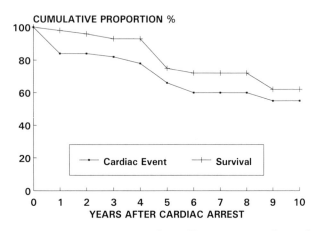

Figure 16. Recurrence rate of cardiac arrest and total survival in 33 survivors of cardiac arrest with hypertrophic cardiomyopathy treated with myomectomy or empiric antiarrhythmic drug therapy. Reproduced with permission from Cecchi F, Maron BJ, Epstein SE. Long-term outcome of patients with hypertrophic cardiomyopathy successfully resuscitated after cardiac arrest. J Am Coll Cardiol 1989;13:1283-1288.

the implantable defibrillator and the patients were managed in a variety of ways. Seventeen underwent septal myectomy and the majority received empiric antiarrhythmic drug therapy. The outcome of a series of such patients when treated with the implantable defibrillator has yet to be published. No clear strategy for the risk assessment of survivors of cardiac arrest in HOCM has been devised. Fananapazir and colleagues[108] performed EPSs in 22 cardiac arrest survivors and found a high rate (77%) of inducible ventricular arrhythmias (polymorphic or monomorphic VT). However, the overall incidence of inducible ventricular arrhythmias in 155 HOCM patients was 43%, and there was no prospective study of the relationship between inducibility and subsequent outcome.

Sustained Monomorphic Ventricular Tachycardia: Spontaneous SMVT occurs in <1% of patients with HOCM, with few cases in the literature.[109,110] In the study by Fananapazir et al,[108] 11% of HOCM patients have inducible monomorphic VT. In two reported cases where it occurred spontaneously, it was associated with left ventricular aneurysm in the presence of normal coronary arteries.[110] Sustained VT was inducible in one of these patients only and both have done well on long-term therapy with amiodarone.

Nonsustained Ventricular Tachycardia: In contrast, NSVT is relatively common in patients with HOCM and may be found in about 25% of adult patients.[111,112] Data from two studies suggest that NSVT is the single best indicator of risk of sudden cardiac death in patients with HOCM.[111,113] Table 5 shows pooled data from these two studies.[114] Patients found to have NSVT on Holter monitoring require further risk stratification, as the positive predictive accuracy for sudden cardiac death is only 22%. The absence of NSVT is of more use as it has a negative predictive accuracy of 97%. Abnormal HRV and abnormal peripheral vasomotor responses are also associated with subsequent sudden cardiac death, although they do not appear to provide any additional prognostic information.[115,116] Empiric amiodarone therapy has been reported to reduce mortality by some[117] but not all[118] groups. Noninvasive techniques such as HRV[119] and signal-averaged ECG[120] have not been shown to improve sensitivity of risk stratification. Detection of fractionated right ventricular electrograms has been noted to be associated with sudden

Table 5

Relation of Nonsustained Ventricular Tachycardia on
Holter Monitoring as a Marker for Risk of Future Sudden
Cardiac Death in 169 Patients with Hypertrophic
Cardiomyopathy

	Sudden Death	
	−	+
NSVT +	9	32
NSVT −	4	124

Sensitivity	69%
Specificity	80%
Prevalence	7.6%
Positive predictive value	22%
Negative predictive value	97%

NSVT: nonsustained ventricular tachycardia. Reproduced with permission from Stewart JT, McKenna WJ: Arrhythmias in hypertrophic cardiomyopathy. J Cardiovasc Electrophysiol 1991; 2:516–524.

cardiac death,[121] but this invasive stratification technique requires prospective evaluation.

In HOCM patients presenting with a cardiac arrest, approximately one of three will suffer a recurrence in the next five years. However, no prospective studies of risk assessment techniques in HOCM cardiac arrest survivors have been performed and the value of invasive EP testing and noninvasive procedures remains uncertain.

Dilated Cardiomyopathy

A number of studies has reported one-year mortality rates for patients with congestive heart failure and New

York Heart Association grade III/IV symptoms to be between 35% and 50%.[122-125] Nearly half of all deaths in patients with congestive heart failure are thought to be of an arrhythmic nature,[126,127] although an unknown proportion of these may be due to bradyarrhythmias.[128,129] In patients without a prior history of ventricular arrhythmias, left ventricular function is a better primary predictor of outcome than conventional Holter monitoring or EPS.[130,131] Three-year survival free of sudden death falls from 92% in patients with an ejection fraction >40% to 71% in patients with an ejection fraction of 30% or less.[130] The signal-averaged ECG has poor sensitivity for identifying patients with ventricular arrhythmias,[132] and the role of HRV remains to be determined.

Two nonrandomized trials of EP-guided drug therapy in patients with dilated cardiomyopathy presenting with ventricular arrhythmias suggest it may be effective at preventing recurrences. In Liem and Swerdlow's study,[133] an effective antiarrhythmic drug therapy was identified in 43% of all patients with inducible sustained ventricular arrhythmia. Survival free of arrhythmia recurrence and sudden cardiac death in these 15 patients at one year was 100%, whereas in the remaining patients, 40% had suffered an arrhythmia recurrence at this stage. In the study by Rae and colleagues,[134] 11 of 25 patients with an inducible ventricular arrhythmia had an antiarrhythmic drug regimen predicted to be effective at EPS. After 21 months (±13 months), follow-up arrhythmia recurrence was 0% in these 11 patients versus 36% in the remainder ($P<0.05$). The role of other risk assessment techniques has yet to be formally evaluated in idiopathic cardiomyopathy patients.

The Cardiomyopathy Trial, a primary trial of the use of the ICD in idiopathic dilated cardiomyopathy patients with a left ventricular ejection fraction of 30% or less and without prior ventricular arrhythmia, is under way.[135] This should extend our knowledge of the natural history of tachyarrhythmias in dilated cardiomyopathy.

Arrhythmogenic Right Ventricular Dysplasia

This cardiomyopathy, which is associated with thinning and aneurysm formation in the right ventricle, may be responsible for up to 50% of VTs of right ventricular origin.[136] The study of prognosis in this group of patients has been limited by the small size of the populations described in many studies. The incidence of cardiac arrest ranges between 0% and 13% at eight years.[137,138] Recurrent episodes of VT, occurring particularly on exercise, are very common, occurring in at least 70% of patients. The majority of arrhythmogenic right ventricular dysplasia patients shows abnormalities of the signal-averaged ECG, but these show considerable variability over time and do not appear to be useful in predicting arrhythmia recurrence and outcome.[139] In addition, inducibility at EPS does not appear to be of use in predicting arrhythmia recurrence.[99,138] The development of progressive right and left ventricular failure may be the most important factor affecting patient outcome.[140]

Chagas' Disease

Between 10 and 20 million South Americans are estimated to have Chagas' disease with a 23% to 30% risk of clinical disease.[141,142] Ventricular arrhythmias are a major cause of death in patients with Chagas' disease,[143] with sudden death occurring in nearly 20% of patients. One study has examined the use of EP-guided drug ther-

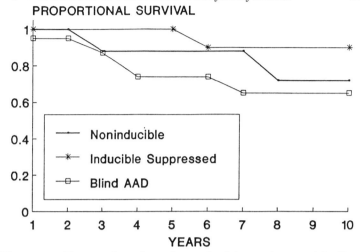

Figure 17. Proportional total survival in patients with Chagas' disease and VT stratified by EPS results. Blind AAD: antiarrhythmic drug therapy not guided by EPS. Reproduced with permission from Giniger AG, Retyk E0, Laino RA, Sananes EG, Lapuente AR. Ventricular tachycardia in Chagas' disease. Am J Cardiol 1992;70:459-462.

apy in patients presenting with symptomatic sustained VT or NSVT.[144] Only 40% of the patients had an inducible arrhythmia and effective therapy was identified in 72% of these patients. There was a trend to better survival in this EP-guided group, although this failed to reach significance (Fig. 17). The role of noninvasive risk assessment in Chagas' disease remains to be evaluated.

Sarcoid

Sarcoidosis is a relatively uncommon cause of sustained VT and, despite cardiac arrhythmias being the lead-

ing cause of death in patients with cardiac sarcoidosis,[145,146] published reports have mostly concerned single
cases or very small series. The largest series[147] consisted
of seven patients, all presenting with hemodynamically
compromising VT with a right bundle branch block pattern. Mean age was 38 years. Clinical VT was induced in
all patients using one or two extrastimuli and a suppressive antiarrhythmic drug regimen was found in five. Despite this, three of the five patients had recurrent VT during an undefined follow-up period. In other case reports,
not all patients have been inducible at EPS.[148,149] These
very limited findings suggest that conventional programmed stimulation may not be very useful in the risk
assessment of patients with sarcoidosis.

Congenital Heart Disease

Surgically repaired congenital heart disease, and particularly tetralogy of Fallot, has been reported to be associated with an increased incidence of ventricular arrhythmias and sudden death in up to 5% of patients.
Increased frequency of ventricular premature beats on
Holter monitoring is associated with subsequent sudden
death[150,151] and also with lower left and right ejection fractions.[152] Inducibility of sustained VT or NSVT at EPS occurs in about 15% of patients and is associated with a history of previous syncope.[153] The signal-averaged ECG has
a sensitivity of 91% and a specificity of 71% in identifying patients with inducible VT at EPS, but did not distin-
guish between those with sustained VT and NSVT.[154]
None of these possible risk assessment techniques has
been applied to the prospective assessment of the risk of
sudden cardiac death in patients with surgically repaired
tetralogy of Fallot.

Discussion

The development of risk assessment techniques for patients with ventricular tachyarrhythmias has made steady progress since the development of invasive EP techniques. However, progress has been limited by the small scale of the many studies that have been conducted. Momentum to improve risk assessment techniques has been stimulated by a number of developments. The more widespread availability of resuscitation techniques has led to an increasing number of cardiac arrest survivors. The realization that the blind use of antiarrhythmic drugs in patients with ventricular extrasystoles could adversely affect survival was emphasized by the results of the Cardiac Arrhythmia Suppression Trial (CAST) study (Fig. 18).[155]

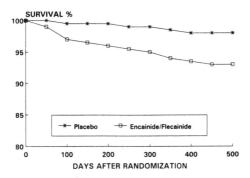

Figure 18. Survival free of death from arrhythmia or cardiac arrest among 1455 patients with prior myocardial infarction and >6 ventricular premature complexes per hour randomized to therapy with placebo, encainide, or flecainide (P = 0.0006). Reproduced with permission from The Cardiac Arrhythmia Suppression Trial (CAST) Investigators. Preliminary report: Effect of encainide and flecainide on mortality in a randomized trial of arrhythmia suppression after myocardial infarction. N Engl J Med 1989;321:406-412.

Finally, the development of the ICD provided a non-pharmacological means to treat ventricular tachyarrhythmias. The relatively high initial cost of the device means that implantation policies based on nonselective use have a relatively poor cost efficacy.[156] The impact of the efficacy and cost of the risk assessment technique used is graphically shown in Figures 19 and 20.

It is clear from the review of risk assessment techniques described above that even for ventricular tachy-

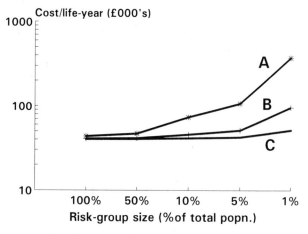

Figure 19. The impact of risk assessment screening test cost on the overall cost efficiency of implantable defibrillator therapy. A: £50 ($75.00); B: £250 ($375.00); C: £1500 ($2250.00). The smaller the high-risk group selected, the more sensitive it is to screening test cost. Reproduced with permission from Anderson MH, Camm AJ. Implications for present and future applications of the implantable cardioverter defibrillator resulting from the use of a simple model of cost-efficacy. Br Heart J 1992;69:83-92.

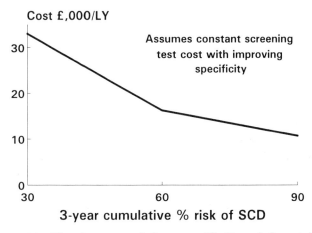

Figure 20. The impact of the specificity of the risk assessment screening test on the overall cost of implantable defibrillator therapy. The higher the untreated cumulative risk of sudden cardiac death (SCD) in the group selected by the screening test, the more cost-effective use of the implantable defibrillator becomes.

arrhythmias associated with coronary artery disease, the scientific application of risk assessment techniques is in its early stages. Invasive EP investigation is a poor primary risk assessment technique as most of its power can be accounted for by differences in left ventricular ejection fraction. It has a more important role in the evaluation of antiarrhythmic drug therapies, provided its limitations are realized. It has yet to be conclusively demonstrated to be superior in this respect to the noninvasive approach using Holter monitoring. For ventricular tachyarrhythmias not associated with underlying coronary artery disease, risk assessment remains primitive because of the small numbers of patients studied.

Future Prospects

The problem of risk assessment of patients with ventricular tachyarrhythmias will only be solved by the results from large, prospective, randomized, and controlled trials of different approaches. Until recently, such trials have received little support because of concerns about the ethical aspects of such studies and the lack of financial incentives for pharmaceutical companies to investigate the use of antiarrhythmic drugs that have patents that may have expired. The development of the implantable defibrillator has had an impact on this situation in two ways. Firstly, it has brought the financial resources of the ICD manufacturers to bear on this problem. Secondly, it has provided a means by which studies of antiarrhythmic drugs may be conducted ethically even with the use of a placebo group, so that patients may be protected from the risk of sudden cardiac death. Such studies are not without their difficulties, however, including the definition of adequate "surrogate end points" in place of sudden death to enable assessment of the results. Nonetheless, the true value of risk assessment techniques in patients with ventricular tachyarrhythmias is likely to become much clearer in the next decade. A fundamental limitation of risk assessment may remain that the occurrence of cardiac arrhythmias, while it may be partly predicted, retains a random element that cannot be identified in advance.

References

1. McWilliam JA. Cardiac failure and sudden death. Br Med J 1889;i:6-8.
2. Gordon T, Kannel WB. Premature mortality from coronary heart disease. The Framingham study. JAMA 1971;215:1617-1625.
3. National Center for Health Statistics. Advance report, final mortality statistics, 1981. Washington, DC: Monthly Vital Statistics Report; 1981. Department of Health and Human Services 33(suppl DHHS):4-5.
4. Thomas A, Knapman P, Krikler D, Davies MJ. Community study of the causes of "natural" sudden death. Br Med J 1988;297:1453-1456.
5. Goldstein S. The necessity of a uniform definition of sudden coronary death: Witnessed death within 1 hour of the onset of acute symptoms. Am Heart J 1982;103:156-159.
6. Hinkle LE, Thaler HT. Clinical classification of cardiac deaths. Circulation 1982;65:457-464.
7. Greene HL, Richardson DW, Barker AH, Roden DM, Capone RJ, Echt DS, et al. Classification of deaths after myocardial infarction as arrhythmic or nonarrhythmic (The Cardiac Arrhythmia Pilot Study). Am J Cardiol 1989;63:1-6.
8. Myerburg RJ, Conde CA, Sung RJ, Mayorga-Cortes A, Mallon SM, Sheps DS, et al. Clinical, electrophysiologic and hemodynamic profile of patients resuscitated from prehospital cardiac arrest. Am J Med 1980;68:568-576.
9. Friedman M, Manwaring JH, Rosenman RH, Donlon G, Ortega P, Grube SM. Instantaneous and sudden deaths. Clinical and pathological differentiations in coronary artery disease. JAMA 1973;225:1319-1328.

10. Liberthson RR, Nagel EL, Hirschman JC, Nussenfeld SR, Blackbourne BD, Davis JH. Pathophysiological observations in prehospital ventricular fibrillation and sudden cardiac death. Circulation 1974;49:790-798.

11. Baum RS, Alvarez H, Cobb LA. Survival after resuscitation from out-of-hospital ventricular fibrillation. Circulation 1974;50:1231-1235.

12. Davies MJ. Anatomic features in victims of sudden coronary death. Circulation 1992;85:I19-I24.

13. Kannel WB, Abbott RD. Incidence and prognosis of unrecognized myocardial infarction: An update on the Framingham study. N Engl J Med 1984;311:1144-1147.

14. Cobbe SM, Redmond MJ, Watson JM, Hollingworth J, Carrington J. "Heartstart Scotland"—initial experience of a national scheme for out-of-hospital defibrillation. Br Med J 1991;302:1517-1520.

15. Cobb LA, Hallstrom AP. Community-based cardiopulmonary resuscitation: What have we learned? Ann NY Acad Sci 1982;382:330-342.

16. Turner AS, Watson OF, Adey HS, Cottle LP, Spence R. The prevalence of disturbance of cardiac rhythm in randomly selected New Zealand adults. New Zealand Med J 1981;93:253-255.

17. Clarke JM, Hamer J, Shelton JR, Taylor S, Venning GR. The rhythm of the normal human heart. Lancet 1976;ii:508-512.

18. Toffler GH, Stone PH, Muller JE, et al. Prognosis after myocardial infarction complicated by ventricular fibrillation. Circulation 1986;74(suppl II):304.

19. Volpi A, Cavalli A, Franzosi MG, Maggioni A, Mauri F, Santoro E. One-year prognosis of primary ventricular fibrillation complicating acute myocardial infarction. Am J Cardiol 1989;63:1174-1178.

20. Kleiman RB, Miller JM, Buxton AE, Josephson ME, Marchlinski FE. Prognosis following sustained ventricular tachycardia occurring early after myocardial infarction. Am J Cardiol 1988;62:528-533.

21. Jensen GV, Torp-Pedersen C, Kober L, Steensgaard-Hansen F, Rasmussen YH, Berning J, et al. Prognosis of late versus early ventricular fibrillation in acute myocardial infarction. Am J Cardiol 1990;66:10-15.

22. Farrell TG, Bashir Y, Cripps T, Malik M, Poloniecki J, Bennett D, et al. Risk stratification for arrhythmic events in postinfarction patients based on heart rate variability, ambulatory electrocardiographic variables and the signal-averaged electrocardiogram. J Am Coll Cardiol 1991;18:687-697.

23. Farrell TG, Odemuyiwa O, Bashir Y, Cripps T, Malik M, Ward DE, et al. Prognostic value of baroreflex sensitivity testing after acute myocardial infarction. Br Heart J 1992;67:129-137.

24. Denniss AR, Richards DA, Cody DV, Russell PA, Yound AA, Ross DL, et al. Prognostic significance of ventricular tachycardia and fibrillation induced at programmed stimulation and delayed potentials detectable on the signal-averaged electrocardiograms of survivors of acute myocardial infarction. Circulation 1986;69:731-745.

25. Liberthson RR, Nagel EL, Hirschman JC, Nussenfeld SR, Blackbourne BD, Davis JH. Pathophysiological observations in prehospital ventricular fibrillation and sudden cardiac death. Circulation 1974;49:790-798.

26. Baum RS, Alvarez H, Cobb LA. Survival after resuscitation from out-of-hospital ventricular fibrillation. Circulation 1974;50:1231-1235.

27. Myerburg RJ, Kessler KM, Estes D, Conde CA, Luceri RM, Zaman L, et al. Long-term survival after pre-

hospital cardiac arrest: Analysis of outcome during an 8 year study. Circulation 1984;70:538-546.

28. Willems AR, Tijssen JGP, van Cappelle FJL, Kingma JH, Hauer RN, Vermeulen FE, et al. Determinants of prognosis in symptomatic ventricular tachycardia or ventricular fibrillation late after myocardial infarction. J Am Coll Cardiol 1990;16:521-530.

29. Josephson ME, Horowitz LN, Farshidi A, Kastor JA. Recurrent sustained ventricular tachycardia. 1. Mechanisms. Circulation 1978;57:431-440.

30. Steurer G, Brugada J, De Bacquer D, Gursoy S, Frey B, Tsakonas K, et al. Value of clinical variables for risk stratification in patients with sustained ventricular tachycardia and history of myocardial infarction. Am J Cardiol 1993;72:349-351.

31. Wilber DJ, Garan H, Finkelstein D, Kelly E, Newell J, McGovern B, et al. Out-of-hospital cardiac arrest. Use of electrophysiological testing in the prediction of long-term survival. N Engl J Med 1988;318:19-24.

32. Mason JW, Swerdlow CD, Winkle RA, Griffin JC, Ross DL, Keefe DL, et al. Programmed ventricular stimulation in predicting vulnerability to ventricular arrhythmias and their response to antiarrhythmic therapy. Am Heart J 1982;103:633-637.

33. Waller TJ, Kay HR, Spielman SR, Kutalek SP, Greenspan AM, Horowitz LN. Reduction in sudden death and total mortality by antiarrhythmic therapy evaluated by electrophysiologic drug testing: Criteria of efficacy in patients with sustained ventricular tachyarrhythmia. J Am Coll Cardiol 1987;10:83-89.

34. Ho DSW, Cooper MJ, Richards DAB, Uther JB, Yip ASB, Ross DL. Comparison of number of extrastimuli versus change in basic cycle length for induction of ventricular tachycardia by programmed ventricu-

lar stimulation. J Am Coll Cardiol 1993;22:1711-1717.

35. McPherson CA, Rosenfeld LE, Batsford WP. Day-to-day reproducibility of responses to right ventricular programmed electrical stimulation: Implications for serial drug testing. Am J Cardiol 1988;62:188-191.

36. Kudenchuk PJ, Kron J, Walance CG, Murphy ES, Morris CD, Griffith KK, et al. Reproducibility of arrhythmia induction with intracardiac electrophysiologic testing: Patients with clinical sustained ventricular tachyarrhythmias. J Am Coll Cardiol 1986;7:819-828.

37. Volgman AS, Zheutlin TA, Mattioni TA, Park MA, Kehoe RF. Reproducibility of programmed electrical stimulation responses in patients with ventricular tachycardia or fibrillation associated with coronary artery disease. Am J Cardiol 1992;70:758-763.

38. Cooper MJ, Koo CC, Skiner MP, Mortensen PT, Hunt LJ, Richards DA, et al. Comparison of immediate versus day to day variability of ventricular tachycardia induction by programmed stimulation. J Am Coll Cardiol 1989;13:1599-1607.

39. Kou WH, de Buitleir M, Kadish AH, Morday F. Sequelae of nonsustained polymorphic ventricular tachycardia induced during programmed ventricular stimulation. Am J Cardiol 1989;64:1148-1151.

40. Wellens HJJ, Brugada P, Stevenson WG. Programmed electrical stimulation of the heart in patients with life-threatening ventricular arrhythmias. What is the significance of induced arrhythmias and what is the correct stimulation protocol? Circulation 1985;72:1-7.

41. Waldo AL, Akhtar M, Brugada P, Henthorn RW, Scheinman MM, Ward DE, et al. The minimally ap-

propriate electrophysiological study for the initial assessment of patients with sustained monomorphic tachycardia. J Am Coll Cardiol 1985;6:1174-1177.

42. Josephson ME. Recurrent ventricular tachycardia. In Clinical Cardiac Electrophysiology: Techniques and Interpretations. Philadelphia: Lea & Fabiger, 1993, pp 417-615.

43. Mason JW, Winkle RA. Accuracy of the ventricular tachycardia-induction study for predicting long-term efficacy and inefficacy of antiarrhythmic drugs. New Engl J Med 1980;303:1073-1077.

44. Ferrick KJ, Luce J, Miller S, Mercando AD, Kim SG, Roth JA, et al. Reproducibility of electrophysiologic testing during antiarrhythmic therapy for ventricular arrhythmias secondary to coronary artery disease. Am J Cardiol 1992;69:1296-1299.

45. Fogoros RN, Elson JJ, Bonnet CA, Fielder SB, Chenarides JG. Reproducibility of successful drug trials in patients with inducible sustained ventricular tachycardia. PACE 1992;15:295-303.

46. Waller TJ, Kay HR, Spielman SR, Kutalek SP, Greenspan AM, Horowitz LN. Reduction in sudden death and total mortality by antiarrhythmic therapy evaluated by electrophysiologic drug testing: Criteria of efficacy in patients with sustained ventricular tachyarrhythmia. J Am Coll Cardiol 1987;10:83-89.

47. Waxman HL, Buxton AE, Sadowski LM, Josephson ME. The response to procainamide during electrophysiologic study for sustained ventricular tachyarrhythmias predicts the response to other medications. Circulation 1983;67:30-37.

48. Kavanagh KM, Wyse G, Duff HJ, Gillis AM, Sheldon RS, Mitchell LB. Drug therapy for ventricular tachyarrhythmias: How many electropharmacological trials are appropriate. J Am Coll Cardiol 1991;17:391-396.

49. Greenspon AJ, Volosin KJ, Greenberg RM, Jefferies L, Rotmensch HH. Amiodarone therapy: Role of early and late electrophysiologic studies. J Am Coll Cardiol 1988;11:117-123.

50. Malois AS, Uricchio F, Mark Estes NA. Prognostic value of early electrophysiologic studies for ventricular tachycardia recurrence in patients with coronary artery disease treated with amiodarone. Am J Cardiol 1989;63:1052-1057.

51. The CASCADE Investigators. Randomized antiarrhythmic drug therapy in survivors of cardiac arrest (the CASCADE Study). Am J Cardiol 1993;72:280-287.

52. The Multicenter Postinfarction Research Group: Risk stratification and survival after myocardial infarction. N Engl J Med 1983;309:331-336.

53. Serruys PW, Simoons ML, Suryapranata H, Vermeer F, Wijns W, van den Brand M, et al. Preservation of global and regional left ventricular function after early thrombolysis in acute myocardial infarction. J Am Coll Cardiol 1986;7:729-742.

54. Levine JH, Mellits D, Baumgardner RA, Veltri EP, Mower M, Grunwald L, et al. Predictors of first discharge and subsequent survival in patients with automatic implantable cardioverter-defibrillators. Circulation 1991;84:558-566.

55. Reiter MJ, Fain ES, Senelly KM. Determinants of recurrent ventricular arrhythmias in patients with implantable pacemaker/defibriliators. Circulation 1991;84:II-426. Abstract.

56. Platia EV, Reid PR. Comparison of programmed electrical stimulation and ambulatory electrocardiographic (Holter) monitoring in the management of ventricular tachycardia and ventricular fibrillation. J Am Coll Cardiol 1984;4:493-500.

57. Skale BT, Miles WM, Heger JJ, Zipes DP, Prystowsky EN. Survivors of cardiac arrest: Prevention of recurrence by drug therapy as predicted by electrophysiologic testing or electrocardiographic monitoring. Am J Cardiol 1986;57:113-119.
58. Mitchell LB, Duff HJ, Manyari DE, Wyse DG. A randomized clinical trial of the noninvasive and invasive approaches to drug therapy of ventricular tachycardia. N Engl J Med 1987;317:1681-1687.
59. The ESVEM Investigators. Determinants of predicted efficacy of antiarrhythmic drugs in the electrophysiologic study versus electrocardiographic monitoring trial. Circulation 1993;87:323-329.
60. Mason JW, for the Electrophysiologic Study versus Electrocardiographic Monitoring Investigators. A comparison of electrophysiologic testing with Holter monitoring to predict antiarrhythmic-drug efficacy for ventricular tachyarrhythmias. N Engl J Med 1993;329:445-451.
61. Bigger JT, Fleiss JL, Kleiger R, Miller JP, Rolnitzky LM. The relationships among ventricular arrhythmias, left ventricular dysfunction and mortality in the 2 years after myocardial infarction. Circulation 1984;69:250-258.
62. Ruberman W, Weinblatt E, Goldberg JD, Frank CW, Chaudhary BS, Shapiro S. Ventricular premature complexes and sudden death after myocardial infarction. Circulation 1981;64:297-305.
63. Bigger JT Jr, Weld FM. Analysis of prognostic significance of ventricular arrhythmias after myocardial infarction: Shortcomings of Lown grading system. Br Heart J 1981;45:717-724.
64. Bigger JT. Relation between left ventricular dysfunction and ventricular arrhythmias after myocardial infarction. Am J Cardiol 1986;57:8B-14B.

65. Farrell TG, Bashir Y, Cripps T, Malik M, Poloniecki J, Bennett D, et al. Risk stratification for arrhythmic events in postinfarction patients based on heart rate variability, ambulatory electrocardiographic variables and the signal-averaged electrocardiogram. J Am Coll Cardiol 1991;18:687-697.

66. Kleiger RE, Miller JP, Bigger JT Jr, Moss AJ. Decreased heart rate variability and its association with increased mortality after acute myocardial infarction. Am J Cardiol 1987;59:256-262.

67. Osterhues HH, Eggeling T, Hoher M, Weismuller P, Kochs M, Hombach V. Value of different non-invasive methods for the recognition of arrhythmogenic complications in high-risk patients with sustained ventricular tachycardia during programmed ventricular stimulation. Eur Heart J 1993;14(suppl E):40-45.

68. Huikuri HV, Valkama JO, Airaksinen J, Seppanen T, Kessler KM, Takkunen JT, et al. Frequency domain measures of heart rate variability before the onset of nonsustained and sustained ventricular tachycardia in patients with coronary artery disease. Circulation 1993;87:1220-1228.

69. Vybirai T, Glaeser DH, Goldberger AL, Rigney DR, Hess KR, Mietus J, et al. Conventional heart rate variability analysis of ambulatory electrocardiographic recordings fails to predict imminent ventricular fibrillation. J Am Coll Cardiol 1993;22:557-565.

70. Simson MB. Use of signals in the terminal QRS complex to identify patients with ventricular tachycardia after myocardial infarction. Circulation 1981; 64:235-241.

71. Breithardt G, Schwarzmaier J, Borggrefe M, Haerten K, Seipel L. Prognostic significance of late ventricular potentials after acute myocardial infarction. Eur Heart J 1983;4:487-495.

72. Gomes JA, Winters SL, Martinson M, Machac J, Stewart D, Targonski A. The prognostic significance of quantitative signal-averaged variables relative to clinical variables, site of myocardial infarction, ejection fraction and ventricular premature beats: A prospective study. J Am Coll Cardiol 1989;13:377-384.

73. Dolack GL, Callahan DB, Bardy GH, Greene HL. Signal averaged electrocardiographic late potentials in resuscitated survivors of out of hospital ventricular fibrillation. Am J Cardiol 1990;65:1102-1104.

74. Epstein AE, Dailey SM, Shepard RB, Kirk KA, Kay GN, Plumb VJ. Inability of signal-averaged electrocardiogram to determine risk of arrhythmia recurrence in patients with implantable cardioverter defibrillators. PACE 1991;14:1169-1178.

75. Sami M, Chaitman B, Fisher L, Holmes D, Fray D, Alderman E. Significance of exercise-induced ventricular arrhythmia in stable coronary artery disease: A coronary artery surgery project. Am J Cardiol 1984;54:1182-1188.

76. Nair CK, Aronow WS, Sketch MH, Pagano T, Lynch JD, Mooss AN, et al. Diagnostic and prognostic significance of exercise-induced premature ventricular complexes in men and women: A four year follow-up. J Am Coll Cardiol 1983;1:1201-1206.

77. Rasmussen K, Lunde PI, Lie M. Coronary bypass surgery in exercise-induced ventricular tachycardia. Eur Heart J 1987;8:444-448.

78. Saini V, Graboys TB, Towne V, Lown B. Reproducibility of exercise-induced ventricular arrhythmia in patients undergoing evaluation for malignant ventricular arrhythmia. Am J Cardiol 1989;63:697-701.

79. Manolis AS, Rastegar H, Mark Estes NA. Effects of coronary artery bypass grafting on ventricular arrhythmias: Results with electrophysiological testing and long-term follow-up. PACE 1993;16:984-991.

80. Anderson KP, DeCamilla J, Moss AJ. Clinical significance of ventricular tachycardia (3 beats or longer) detected during ambulatory monitoring after myocardial infarction. Circulation 1978;57:890-897.

81. Bigger JT, Weld FM, Rolnitzky LM. Prevalence, characteristics and significance of ventricular tachycardia (3 or more complexes) detected with ambulatory electrocardiographic recording in the late hospital phase of acute myocardial infarction. Am J Cardiol 1981;48:815-823.

82. Kleiger RE, Miller JP, Thanavaro S, Province MA, Martin TF, Oliver GC. Relationship between ciinical features of acute myocardial infarction and ventricular runs 2 weeks to 1 year after myocardial infarction. Circulation 1978;57:890-897.

83. Pratt CM, Hallstrom A, Theroux P, Romhilt D, Coromilas J, Myles J. Avoiding pitfalls when assessing arrhythmia suppression after myocardial infarction: Insights from the long-term observations of the placebo-treated patients in the Cardiac Arrhythmia Pilot Study (CAPS). J Am Coll Cardiol 1991;17:1-8.

84. Turrito G, Fontaine JM, Ursell S, Caref EB, Bekheit S, El-Sherif N. Risk stratification and management of patients with organic heart disease and nonsustained ventricular tachycardia: Role of programmed stimulation, left ventricular ejection fraction and signal-averaged electrocardiogram. Am J Med 1990;88:35N-41N.

85. Hammill SC, Trusty JM, Wood DL, Bailey KR, Vatterot PJ, Osborn MJ, et al. Influence of ventricular

function and presence or absence of coronary artery disease on results of electrophysiologic testing for asymptomatic nonsustained ventricular tachycardia. Am J Cardiol 1990;65:722-728.

86. Kowey PR, Waxman HL, Greenspon A, Greenberg R, Poll D, Kutalek S, et al. Philadelphia Arrhythmia Group. Value of electrophysiologic testing in patients with previous myocardial infarction and nonsustained ventricular tachycardia. Am J Cardiol 1990;65:594-598.

87. Wilber DJ, Olshansky B, Moran JF, Scanlon PJ. Electrophysiological testing and nonsustained ventricular tachycardia. Circulation 1990;82:350-358.

88. Manolis AS, Estes NA. Value of programmed ventricular stimulation in the evaluation and management of patients with nonsustained ventricular tachycardia associated with coronary artery disease. Am J Cardiol 1990;65:201-205.

89. Klein-RC, Machell-C. Use of electrophysiologic testing in patients with nonsustained ventricular tachycardia: Prognostic and therapeutic implications. J Am Coll Cardiol 1989;14:155-161.

90. Kowey PR, Taylor JE, Marinchak RA, Rials SJ. Does programmed stimulation really help in the evaluation of patients with nonsustained ventricular tachycardia? Results of a meta-analysis. Am Heart J 1992;123:481-485.

91. Buxton AE, Fisher JD, Josephson ME, Lee KL, Pryor DB, Prystowsky EN, et al. Prevention of sudden death in patients with coronary artery disease: The Multicenter Unsustained Tachycardia Trial (MUSTT). Prog Cardiovasc Dis 1993;36:215-226.

92. MADIT Executive Committee: Multicenter automatic defibrillator implantation trial (MADIT): Design and clinical protocol. PACE 1991;14:920-927.

93. Winters SL, Stewart D, Targonski A, Gomes JA. Role of signal averaging of the surface QRS complex in selecting patients with nonsustained ventricular tachycardia and high grade ventricular arrhythmias for programmed ventricular stimulation. J Am Coll Cardiol 1988;12:1481-1487.

94. Turitto G, Fontaine JM, Ursell SN, Caref EB, Henkin R, El-Sherif N. Value of the signal-averaged electrocardiogram as a predictor of the results of programmed stimulation in non-sustained ventricular tachycardia. Am J Cardiol 1988;61:1272-1278.

95. Nava A, Thiene G, Canciani B, Martini B, Daliento L, Buja G, et al. Clinical profile of concealed form of arrhythmogenic right ventricular cardiomyopathy presenting with apparently idiopathic ventricular arrhythmias. Int J Cardiol 1992;35:195-206.

96. Gill JS, Hunter GJ, Gane J, Ward DE, Camm AJ. Asymmetry of cardiac [123I] meta-iodobenzyl-guanidine scans in patients with ventricular tachycardia and "clinically normal" heart. Br Heart J 1993;69:6-13.

97. Mont L, Seixas T, Brugada P, Brugada J, Simonis F, Kriek E, et al. The electrocardiographic, clinical, and electrophysiologic spectrum of idiopathic monomorphic ventricular tachycardia. Am Heart J 1992; 124:746-753.

98. Okumura K, Matsuyama K, Miyagi H, Tsuchiya T, Yasue H. Entrainment of idiopathic ventricular tachycardia of left ventricular origin with evidence for reentry with an area of slow conduction and effect of verapamil. Am J Cardiol 1988;62:727-732.

99. Lemery R, Brugada P, Bella PD, Dugernier T, van den Dool A, Wellens HJJ. Nonischemic ventricular tachycardia: Clinical course and long-term follow-up in patients without clinically overt heart disease. Circulation 1989;79:990-999.

100. Yamamoto K, Bando S, Nishikado A, Ikefuji H, Shinohara A, Ito S. Two sudden death cases of idiopathic ventricular tachycardia. Tokushima J Exp Med 1992;39:127-134.

101. Coggins DL, Lee RJ, Sweeney J, Chein WW, Van Hare G, Epstein L, et al. Radiofrequency catheter ablation as a cure for idiopathic tachycardia of both left and right ventricular origin. J Am Coll Cardiol 1994;23:1333-1341.

102. Mehta D, Camm AJ. Signal-averaged electrocardiography and the significance of late potentials in patients with idiopathic ventricular tachycardia: A review. Clin Cardiol 1989;12:307-312.

103. Fei L, Anderson MH, Katritsis D, Sneddon J, Statter DJ, Malik M, et al. Decreased heart rate variability in survivors of sudden cardiac death not associated with coronary artery disease. Br Heart J 1994;71:16-21.

104. Chandra NC, Gates EA, Thamer M. Conservative treatment of paroxysmal ventricular tachycardia during pregnancy. Clin Cardiol 1991;14:347-350.

105. McKenna WJ. The natural history of hypertrophic cardiomyopathy. Cardiovasc Clin 1988;19:135-148.

106. Nicod P, Polikar R, Peterson KL. Hypertrophic cardiomyopathy and sudden death. New Engl J Med 1988;318:1255-1256.

107. Cecchi F, Maron BJ, Epstein SE. Long-term outcome of patients with hypertrophic cardiomyopathy successfully resuscitated after cardiac arrest. J Am Coll Cardiol 1989;13:1283-1288.

108. Fananapazir L, Tracy CM, Leon MB, Winkler JB, Cannon RO, Bonow RO, et al. Electrophysiologic abnormalities in patients with hypertrophic cardiomyopathy. A consecutive analysis in 155 patients. Circulation 1989;80:1259-1268.

109. Geibel A, Brugada P, Zehender M, Stevenson W, Waldecker B, Wellens HJ. Value of programmed electrical stimulation using a standardized ventricular stimulation protocol in hypertrophic cardiomyopathy. Am J Cardiol 1987;60:738-739.
110. Alfonso F, Frenneaux M, McKenna WJ. Clinical sustained uniform ventricular tachycardia in hypertrophic cardiomyopathy: Association with left ventricular apical aneurysm. Br Heart J 1989;61: 178-181.
111. McKenna WJ, England D, Doi YL, Deanfield JE, Oakley CE, Goodwin JF. Arrhythmia in hypertrophic cardiomyopathy. 1. Influence on prognosis. Br Heart J 1981;46:168-172.
112. Savage DD, Seides SF, Maron BJ, Myers DJ, Epstein SE. Prevalence of arrhythmia during 24-hour electrocardiographic monitoring and exercise testing in patients with obstructive and non-obstructive hypertrophic cardiomyopathy. Circulation 1979;59: 866-875.
113. Maron BJ, Savage DD, Wolfson JK, Epstein SE. Prognostic significance of 24-hour ambulatory electrocardiographic monitoring in patients with hypertrophic cardiomyopathy. A prospective study. Am J Cardiol 1981;48:252-257.
114. Stewart JT, McKenna WJ. Arrhythmias in hypertrophic cardiomyopathy. J Cardiovasc Electrophysiol 1991;2:516-524.
115. Counihan PJ, Fie L, Bashir Y, Farrell TG, Haywood GA, McKenna WJ. Assessment of heart rate variability in hypertrophic cardiomyopathy. Circulation 1993;88:1682-1690.
116. Counihan PJ, Haywood GA, Webb DJ, McKenna WJ. Abnormal vascular responses during supine exer-

cise in hypertrophic cardiomyopathy. Circulation 1991;84:686-696.

117. McKenna WJ, Oakley CM, Krikler DM, Goodwin JF. Improved survival with amiodarone in patients with hypertrophic cardiomyopathy and ventricular tachycardia. Br Heart J 1985;53:412-416.

118. Fananapazir L, Leon MB, Bonow RO, Tracy CM, Cannon RO, Epstein SE. Sudden death during empiric amiodarone therapy in symptomatic hypertrophic cardiomyopathy. Am J Cardiol 1991;67:169-175.

119. Counihan PJ, Lu F, Bashir Y, Farrell TG, Haywood GA, McKenna WJ. Assessment of heart rate variability in hypertrophic cardiomyopathy. Circulation 1993;88:1682-1690.

120. Kulakowski P, Counihan PJ, Camm AJ, McKenna WJ. The value of time and frequency domain, and spectral temporal mapping analysis of the signal-averaged electrocardiogram in identification of patients with hypertrophic cardiomyopathy at increased risk of sudden death. Eur Heart J 1993;14:941-950.

121. Saumarez RC, Camm AJ, Panagos A, Gill JS, Stewart JT, de Belder MA, et al. Ventricular fibrillation in hypertrophic cardiomyopathy is associated with increased fractionation of paced right ventricular electrograms. Circulation 1992;86:467-474.

122. The CONSENSUS Trial Study Group. Effects of enalapril on mortality in severe congestive heart failure. N Engl J Med 1987;316:432-447.

123. Chatterjee K, Parmley WW, Cohn JN, Levine TB, Awan NA, Mason DT, et al. A cooperative multicenter study of captopril in congestive heart failure: Haemodynamic effects and long term responses. Am Heart J 1985;110:439-447.

124. King J, Steingo L, Barlow JB, Jardine R, Goldman AP, Allman B, et al. Further experience with long-term

captopril therapy in severe refractory congestive cardiac heart failure. SA Med J 1983;64:510-515.

125. Kao W, Gheorghiade M, Hall V, Goldstein S. Relation between plasma norepinephrine and response to medical therapy in men with congestive heart failure secondary to coronary artery disease or idiopathic dilated cardiomyopathy. Am J Cardiol 1989;64:609-613.

126. Packer M. Sudden unexpected death in patients with congestive heart failure: A second frontier. Circulation 1985;72:681-685.

127. Francis G. Should asymptomatic ventricular arrhythmias in patients with congestive heart failure be treated with antiarrhythmic drugs? J Am Coll Cardiol 1988;12:274-276.

128. Ando S, Koyanagi S, Muramatsu K, Itaya R, Takeshita A, Nakamura M. Clinical characteristics of patients with dilated cardiomyopathy and bradyarrhythmias. J Cardiol 1991;21:53-91.

129. Radhakrishnan S, Kaul U, Bahl VK, Talwar KK, Bhatia ML. Sudden bradyarrhythmic death in dilated cardiomyopathy: A case report. PACE 1988;11:1369-1372.

130. Olshausen KV, Stienen U, Schwarz F, Kubler W, Meyer JSO. Long-term prognostic significance of ventricular arrhythmias in idiopathic dilated cardiomyopathy. Am J Cardiol 1988;61:146-151.

131. Kron J, Hart M, Schual-Berke S, Niles NR, Hosenpud JD, McAnulty JH. Idiopathic dilated cardiomyopathy. Role of programmed electrical stimulation and Holter monitoring in predicting those at risk of sudden death. Chest 1988;93:85-90.

132. Keeling PJ, Kulakowski P, Yi G, Slade AKB, Bent SE, McKenna WJ. Usefulness of signal-averaged electrocardiogram in idiopathic dilated cardiomyopathy

for identifying patients with ventricular arrhythmias. Am J Cardiol 1993;72:78-84.

133. Liem LB, Swerdlow CD. Value of electropharmacologic testing in idiopathic dilated cardiomyopathy and sustained ventricular tachyarrhythmias. Am J Cardiol 1988;62:611-616.

134. Rae AP, Spielman SR, Kutalek SP, Kay HR, Horowitz LN. Electrophysiologic assessment of antiarrhythmic drug efficacy for ventricular tachyarrhythmias associated with dilated cardiomyopathy. Am J Cardiol 1987;59:291-295.

135. The Cardiomyopathy Trial Investigators. Cardiomyopathy trial. PACE 1993;16:576-581.

136. Lesaka Y, Hiroe M, Aonuma K, Nitta J, Nogami A, Tokunaga T, et al. Usefulness of electrophysiologic study and endomyocardial biopsy in differentiating arrhythmogenic right ventricular dysplasia from idiopathic right ventricular tachycardia. Heart Vessels 1990;5(suppl):65-69.

137. Blomstrom-Lundqvist C, Sabel KG, Olsson SB. A long term follow up of 15 patients with arrhythmogenic right ventricular dysplasia. Br Heart J 1987;58:477-488.

138. Lemery R, Brugada P, Janssen J, Cheriex E, Dugernier T, Wellens HJ. Nonischemic sustained ventricular tachycardia: Clinical outcome in 12 patients with arrhythmogenic right ventricular dysplasia. J Am Coll Cardiol 1989;14:96-105.

139. Blomstrom-Lundqvist C, Olsson SB, Edvardsson N. Follow-up by repeated signal-averaged surface QRS in patients with the syndrome of arrhythmogenic right ventricular dysplasia. Eur Heart J 1989;10(suppl D):54-60.

140. Leclercq JF, Coumel P. Characteristics, prognosis and treatment of the ventricular arrhythmias of right ventricular dysplasia. Eur Heart J 1989;10:61-67.

141. Laraja FS, Dias E, Nobrega G, Miranda A. Chagas' disease: A clinical epidemiological and pathological study. Circulation 1956;14:1035-1060.
142. World Health Organization. Chagas' disease. Sixth report of the scientific group on Chagas' disease. 1982.
143. Chiale PA, Halpern MS, Nau GJ, Przybylski J, Tambussi AM, Lazzari JO, et al. Malignant ventricular arrhythmias in chronic chagasic myocarditis. PACE 1982;5:162-172.
144. Giniger AG, Retyk EO, Laino RA, Sananes EG, Lapuente AR. Ventricular tachycardia in Chagas' disease. Am J Cardiol 1992;70:459-462.
145. Roberts WC, McAllister HA, Ferrans VJ. Sarcoidosis of the heart. A clinicopathologic study of 35 necropsy patients (group I) and review of 78 previously described necropsy patients (group II). Am J Med 1977;63:86-108.
146. Stein E, Stimmel B, Slitzbach LE. Clinical course of cardiac sarcoidosis. Ann NY Acad Sci 1976;278:470-474.
147. Winters SL, Cohen M, Greenberg S, Stein B, Curwin J, Pe E, et al. Sustained ventricular tachycardia associated with sarcoidosis: Assessment of the underlying cardiac anatomy and the prospective utility of programmed ventricular stimulation, drug therapy and an implantable antitachycardia device. J Am Coll Cardiol 1991;18:937-943.
148. Bharati S, Lev M, Denes P, Modlinger J, Wyndham C, Bauernfeind R, et al. Infiltrative cardiomyopathy with conduction disease and ventricular arrhythmias: Electrophysiologic and pathologic correlations. Am J Cardiol 1980;45:163-173.
149. Morady F, Scheinman MM, Hess DS, Chen R, Stanger P. Clinical characteristics and results of electro-

physiologic testing in young adults with ventricular tachycardia or ventricular fibrillation. Am Heart J 1985;106:1306-1314.

150. Gillette PC, Yeoman MA, Mullins CE, McNamara DG. Sudden death after repair of tetralogy of Fallot. Electrocardiographic and electrophysiologic abnormalities. Circulation 1977;56:566-571.

151. Kavey RE, Blackman MS, Sondheimer HM. Incidence and severity of chronic ventricular dysrhythmias after repair of tetralogy of Fallot. Am Heart J 1982;103:342-350.

152. Kavey RE, Thomas FD, Byrum CJ, Blackman MS, Sondheimer HM, Bove EL. Ventricular arrhythmias and biventricular dysfunction after repair of tetralogy of Fallot. J Am Coll Cardiol 1984;4:126-131.

153. Garson A Jr, Porter CB, Gillette PC, McNamara DG. Induction of ventricular tachycardia during electrophysiologic study after repair of tetralogy of Fallot. J Am Coll Cardiol 1983;1:1493-1502.

154. Stelling JA, Danford DA, Kugler JD, Windle JR, Cheatham JP, Gumbiner CH, et al. Late potentials and inducible ventricular tachycardia in surgically repaired congenital heart disease. Circulation 1990; 82:1690-1696.

155. The Cardiac Arrhythmia Suppression Trial (CAST) Investigators. Preliminary report: Effect of encainide and flecainide on mortality in a randomized trial of arrhythmia suppression after myocardial infarction. N Engl J Med 1989;321:406-412.

156. Anderson MH, Camm AJ. Implications for present and future applications of the implantable cardioverter defibrillator resulting from the use of a simple model of cost-efficacy. Br Heart J 1992;69:83-92.

Index